GREAT LIFE

Unlocking the astonishing connection between metabolism and optimal health

Alyssa Anderson

GREAT LIFE

GREAT LIFE

GREAT LIFE

GREAT LIFE

GREAT LIFE

INTRODUCTION

Characterizing Extraordinary Energy

Human energy prerequisites are assessed from proportions of energy use in addition to the extra energy needs for development, pregnancy and lactation. Proposals for dietary energy admission from food should fulfill these prerequisites for the achievement and upkeep of ideal wellbeing, physiological capability and prosperity. The last option (for example prosperity) depends on wellbeing, yet in addition on the capacity to fulfill the requests forced by society and the climate, as well as the wide range of various energy-requesting exercises that satisfy individual requirements.

GREAT LIFE

Energy balance is accomplished when input (for example dietary energy admission) is equivalent to yield (for example all out energy use), in addition to the energy cost of development in youth and pregnancy, or the energy cost to deliver milk during lactation. At the point when energy balance is kept up with over a delayed period, an individual is viewed as in a consistent state. This can incorporate brief periods during which the everyday harmony among admission and use doesn't happen. An ideal consistent state is accomplished when energy consumption makes up for all out energy use and considers satisfactory development in kids, and pregnancy and lactation in ladies, without forcing metabolic, physiological or

GREAT LIFE

conduct limitations that limit the full articulation of an individual's natural, social and financial potential.

Inside specific cutoff points, people can adjust to transient or getting through changes in energy admission through conceivable physiological and social reactions connected with energy consumption or potentially changes in development. Energy balance is kept up with, and another consistent state is then accomplished. Notwithstanding, acclimations to low or high energy admissions may once in a while involve natural and conduct punishments, for example, decreased development speed, loss of lean weight, exorbitant collection of muscle versus fat, expanded chance of illness, constrained rest periods, and physical

GREAT LIFE

or social impediments in playing out specific exercises and errands. A portion of these changes are significant and may try and expand the possibilities of endurance in the midst of food shortage.

A sufficient, solid eating regimen should fulfill human requirements for energy and every single fundamental supplement. Moreover, dietary energy needs and proposals can't be viewed as in seclusion of different supplements in the eating routine, as the absence of one will impact the others. In this manner, the accompanying definitions depend with the understanding that prerequisites for energy will be satisfied through the utilization of an eating routine that fulfills every supplement need. Energy prerequisite is

GREAT LIFE

how much food energy expected to adjust energy use to keep up with body size, body organization and a degree of fundamental and beneficial actual work steady with long haul great wellbeing. This incorporates the energy required for the ideal development and advancement of youngsters, for the affidavit of tissues during pregnancy, and for the discharge of milk during lactation predictable with the great soundness of mother and kid. The suggested degree of dietary energy consumption for a populace bunch is the mean energy necessity of the sound, very much sustained people who comprise that gathering.

In light of these definitions, a fundamental target for the evaluation of energy prerequisites is the solution of

GREAT LIFE

dietary energy admissions that are viable with long haul great wellbeing. Thusly, the degrees of energy consumption suggested by this master meeting depend on evaluations of the prerequisites of sound, very much fed people. It is perceived that a few populaces have specific general wellbeing qualities that are important for their standard thing, "ordinary" life. First among these are populace bunches in many emerging nations where there are various babies and youngsters who experience the ill effects of gentle to direct levels of lack of healthy sustenance and who experience continuous episodes of irresistible sicknesses, for the most part diarrhoeal and respiratory contaminations.

GREAT LIFE

Extraordinary contemplations are made in this report for such sub-populaces.

The Significance of Digestion in Wellbeing

You might have heard the terms digestion, metabolic rate and basal metabolic rate utilized reciprocally. They generally mean marginally various things, so here's an outline:

Digestion

Digestion alludes to the substance processes that occur as your body changes over food and drink into energy. The cycle consolidates calories with oxygen to deliver energy. This fills significant cycles like:

Relaxing

GREAT LIFE

Directing your internal heat level

Processing food

Delivering pee

Circling blood

Fixing harmed tissues

Overseeing chemical levels

Metabolic rate

Metabolic rate is one part of the metabolic interaction - it's the speed or recurrence of your digestion. The basal metabolic rate (BMR) is the base number of calories your body needs to work while resting. Everybody's BMR is unique, yet overall, men need around 2,500

GREAT LIFE

calories and ladies need around 2,000 calories each day to keep up with their weight.

There are 3 principal ways your body consumes energy consistently:

The basal digestion - the energy your body uses to work while very still. This incorporates energy expected to breath, flow blood and cell creation among others

The energy you use to separate food (otherwise called the thermic impact)

The energy you use during actual work

It merits recalling that the vast majority of the energy you consume is from your resting digestion - around 75%.

GREAT LIFE

What influences your metabolic rate?

The capability and speed of your digestion is impacted by bunches of various things, and it changes from one individual to another. The key variables include:

Bulk - individuals with more bulk typically have a quicker digestion

Age - age doesn't influence digestion all alone however, with age, bulk will in general decrease while diet continues as before

Organic sex - men typically have a quicker metabolic rate since they will quite often be huge than ladies

Chemical issues - an underactive thyroid for instance can make you have a more slow digestion

GREAT LIFE

Regular body size and fat piece

Hereditary qualities - researchers are as yet attempting to figure out this yet we really do realize that certain individuals can foster muscle more straightforward than others

Strangely, the feminine cycle likewise assumes a minor part. Research has found that a few ladies have a higher metabolic rate during the last 50% of their period, while the resting metabolic rate for certain ladies depends on 10% higher.

Digestion as a matter of fact is the expenditure of calories by the body to get the energy expected for the body. Metabolic rate relies upon the age, orientation, fat

GREAT LIFE

and bulk of the body, action level and a little on hereditary variables. Just hereditary among these elements may not be changed. The remainder rely upon the individual as it were. The pace of expenditure calories, that is the metabolic rate, can be changed with straightforward and little changes.

Techniques to Speed up the Digestion

Standard eating: Eating at specific times consistently can help keeping up with the metabolic equilibrium. Customary eating can be considered as the initial step to arrive at the objective of expanding the metabolic rate.

GREAT LIFE

Adequate calory admission: Consuming unsuitable feasts can have same activity with indulging. Too little calory admission can make dialing back of digestion conserve in energy.

Performing Strength Preparing: Strength preparing for working out assists with creating muscles. The bulk has a higher metabolic rate when contrasted with fat, or at least, keeping up with the bulk requires more energy when contrasted with fat. Individual lose their muscles with age. Normal strength preparing will expand the bulk, and thus, digestion will speed up.

To drink adequate measures of water: Keeping up with the liquid equilibrium of the body is vital as respects the right activity of essential capabilities and forestalling

GREAT LIFE

the dialing back of metabolic rate. Drinking adequate measures of water can assist with getting in shape. A few examinations have shown that body loads and weight records in overweight ladies who increment their everyday water utilization to 1,5 liters.

To diminish pressure: Stress influences the chemical levels and can cause creation of cortisol more than ordinary. Cortisol is a chemical that manages hunger. In view of studies, cortisol creation in over the top sums can bring about weight gain and subsequently, expansion in the metabolic rate.

Extreme focus Working out: Extreme focus discontinuous working out (HIIT) can accelerate the digestion like strength preparing. That is, focused

GREAT LIFE

energy irregular activity following strength preparing will both decidedly influence the metabolic rate and help getting thinner.

Sleeping: Having sufficient rest can assist with keeping up with the equilibrium of chemicals, and along these lines, you won't eat a lot. While the quantity of long periods of rest required changes among people, concentrates on show that grown-ups need no less than 7 to 8 hours of rest day to day.

GREAT LIFE

GREAT LIFE

CHAPTER ONE
FIGURING OUT DIGESTION

Outline of Metabolic Cycles

What's happening in your body at the present time? Your most memorable response may be that you're ravenous, or that your muscles are sore from a run, or that you feel tired. Be that as it may, we should go considerably more profound, moving past the layer of your cognizance and seeing what's going in your cells.

On the off chance that you could look within any cell in your body, you'd observe that it was an exceptional center of action, more like a bustling outside market than a tranquil room. Whether you are alert or dozing,

GREAT LIFE

running or staring at the television, energy is being changed inside your phones, changing structures as particles go through the associated substance responses that keep you alive and useful. Cells are continually doing huge number of synthetic responses expected to keep the cell, and your body overall, alive and sound. These substance responses are in many cases connected together in chains, or pathways. Each of the synthetic responses that happen within a phone are on the whole called the phone's digestion. To get a feeling of the intricacy of digestion, we should investigate the metabolic outline underneath. As far as I might be concerned, this wreck of lines seems to be a guide of an extremely enormous tram framework, or conceivably an

GREAT LIFE

extravagant circuit board. Truth be told, it's a graph of the center metabolic pathways in an eukaryotic cell, like the cells that make up the human body. Each line is a response, and each circle is a reactant or item. In the metabolic trap of the cell, a portion of the compound responses discharge energy and can happen immediately (without energy input). In any case, others need added energy to occur. Similarly as you should persistently eat food to supplant what your body utilizes, so cells need a ceaseless inflow of energy to drive their energy-requiring substance responses. As a matter of fact, the food you eat is the wellspring of the energy utilized by your phones!

GREAT LIFE

To make the possibility of digestion more concrete, we should take a gander at two metabolic cycles that are urgent to life on the planet: those that form sugars, and those that separate them.

Separating glucose: Cell breath

To act as an illustration of an energy-delivering pathway, we should perceive how one of your phones could separate a sugar particle (say, from that treats you had for dessert).

Numerous phones, including the majority of the phones in your body, get energy from glucose in a cycle called cell breath. During this cycle, a glucose particle is

GREAT LIFE

separated continuously, in many little advances. Nonetheless, the cycle has a general response of:

Separating glucose discharges energy, which is caught by the cell as adenosine triphosphate, or ATP. ATP is a little particle that gives cells a helpful approach to store energy momentarily.

Whenever it's made, ATP can be involved by different responses in the cell as an energy source. Much as we people use cash since it's simpler than dealing each time we really want something, so the cell utilizes ATP to have a normalized method for moving energy. Along these lines, ATP is once in a while portrayed as the "energy cash" of the cell.

GREAT LIFE

Developing glucose: Photosynthesis

To act as an illustration of an energy-requiring metabolic pathway, we should flip that last model around and perceive how a sugar particle is fabricated.

Sugars like glucose are made by plants in a cycle called photosynthesis. In photosynthesis, plants utilize the energy of daylight to change over carbon dioxide gas into sugar atoms. Photosynthesis happens in many little advances, however its general response is only the cell breath response flipped in reverse:

Like us, plants need energy to drive their cell processes, so a portion of the sugars are utilized by the actual plant. They can likewise give a food source to creatures

GREAT LIFE

that eat the plant, similar to the squirrel beneath. In the two cases, the glucose will be separated through cell breath, creating ATP to keep cells running.

Factors Impacting Digestion

To remain alive and working, your body needs to complete huge number of compound cycles, which are all things considered known as your digestion.

Your digestion can assume a part in weight gain by impacting how much energy your body needs at some random point. Abundance energy is then put away as fat.

Try not to rush to fault a 'inability to burn calories' for weight gain as better food decisions and exercise have the greatest effect.

GREAT LIFE

The greatest part of your digestion, (50-80%) of the energy utilized, is your basal metabolic rate (BMR), which is the energy your body consumes just to keep up with working very still.

The following are ten factors that influence BMR and digestion:

Bulk. How much muscle tissue on your body. Working muscle takes more energy than working fat. So the more muscle tissue you convey, the more energy your body needs to exist.

This rundown shows us that a few things you can change to modify your BMR and a few things you can't.

GREAT LIFE

Fortunately you can do a lot to change the equilibrium. (Obstruction or strength preparing is best for building and keeping up with mass.)

Age. As you progress in years, your metabolic rate for the most part eases back. This is a result of a deficiency of muscle tissue and changes to hormonal and neurological cycles. During improvement kids go through times of development with outrageous paces of digestion.

Body size. Those with greater bodies have a bigger BMR since they have bigger organs and liquid volume to keep up with.

GREAT LIFE

Gender. Men for the most part have quicker digestion systems than ladies.

Genetics. A few families have quicker BMR than others for certain hereditary problems likewise influencing digestion.

Actual work. Practice increments bulk and powers up your metabolic motors consuming kilojoules at a quicker rate, in any event, when very still.

Hormonal variables. Hormonal irregular characteristics like hypo and hyperthyroidism can influence your digestion.

Ecological variables. Natural changes, for example, expanded intensity or cold powers the body to work harder to keep up with its generally expected temperature and builds BMR.

Drugs. Caffeine and nicotine can build your BMR while prescriptions, for example, antidepressants and steroids increment weight gain paying little mind to what you eat.

Diet. Food changes your digestion. What and how you eat affects your BMR.

This once-over shows us that a couple of things you can change to alter your BMR and a couple of things you can't. Thankfully, you can significantly alter the equilibrium. Chiropractic standards let us know that attempting to make a body that functions admirably

GREAT LIFE

without obstruction will intensely influence wellbeing. The food, exercise and movement decisions that we make can likewise build BMR and diminish obstruction to the sensory system permitting your body to flourish. A mutually beneficial arrangement.

GREAT LIFE

GREAT LIFE

GREAT LIFE

CHAPTER TWO
THE CONNECTION AMONG DIGESTION AND WELLBEING

Digestion and Weight The board

Certain individuals put their weight on how their body separates food into energy, otherwise called digestion. They think their digestion is excessively sluggish. However, is that actually the reason? Provided that this is true, is it conceivable to accelerate the cycle?

The facts confirm that the rate at which the body separates food is connected to weight. Be that as it may, an inability to burn calories isn't normally the reason for weight gain.

GREAT LIFE

Digestion concludes how much energy a body needs. Be that as it may, weight relies heavily on how much an individual eats and beverages joined with actual work.

Metabolism: Changing over food into energy

Digestion is the cycle by which the body changes food and drink into energy. During this cycle, calories in food and refreshments mix in with oxygen to make the energy the body needs. To be sure, even exceptionally still, a body needs energy for all it does. This integrates breathing, sending blood through the body, keeping synthetic levels even, and creating and fixing cells. The quantity of calories a body very still purposes to do these things is known as basal metabolic rate, likewise called basal digestion.

GREAT LIFE

Bulk is the primary calculate basal metabolic rate. Basal metabolic rate additionally relies upon:

Body size and creation. Individuals who are bigger or have more muscle consume more calories, even very still.

Sex. Men normally have less muscle versus fat and more muscle than do ladies of a similar age and weight. That implies men consume more calories.

Age. With maturing, individuals will more often than not lose muscle. A greater amount of the body's weight is from fat, which eases back calorie consuming.

GREAT LIFE

Other than the basal metabolic rate, two different things conclude the number of calories a body that consumes every day:

How the body utilizes food. Processing, retaining, moving and putting away food consume calories. Around 10% of calories eaten are utilized for processing food and taking in supplements. This can't be changed a lot.

How much a body moves. Any turn of events, such as playing tennis, walking around a store or chasing after the canine, makes up different calories a body consumes consistently. This can be changed a ton, both by doing more activity and simply moving really during the day.

GREAT LIFE

Day to day movement that isn't practice is called nonexercise action thermogenesis (Flawless). This incorporates strolling around the house. It additionally incorporates exercises like cultivating and housework, and in any event, squirming. Perfect records for around 100 to 800 calories utilized everyday.

Digestion and weight

You should fault an ailment for inability to burn calories and weight gain. In any case, seldom does an ailment sub-optimal ability to burn calories enough to cause a ton of weight gain. Conditions that can cause weight gain incorporate Cushing disorder or having an underactive thyroid organ, otherwise called hypothyroidism. These circumstances are phenomenal.

GREAT LIFE

Numerous things influence weight gain. These logical incorporate qualities, chemicals, diet and way of life, including rest, active work and stress. You put on weight when you eat a greater number of calories than you consume — or consume less calories than you eat.

Certain individuals appear to get in shape more rapidly and more effectively than others. In any case, everybody gets thinner by consuming a larger number of calories than are eaten. The reality is calories count. To shed pounds, you want to eat less calories or consume actual work. Then again you can do both.

A more intensive gander at active work and digestion

GREAT LIFE

You can only with significant effort control the speed of your basal metabolic rate, yet you have some control over the number of calories you that consume active work. The more dynamic you are, the more calories you consume. As a matter of fact, certain individuals who appear to have a quick digestion are likely more dynamic — and perhaps squirm more — than others.

To consume more calories, the Dynamic work Rules for Americans proposes the going with:

Vigorous movement. As an overall objective, hold back nothing 30 minutes of moderate active work consistently. To get in shape, keep up with weight reduction or meet explicit wellness objectives, you might have to practice more. Moderate oxygen

GREAT LIFE

consuming activity incorporates exercises like energetic strolling, trekking, swimming and cutting the grass. Fiery oxygen consuming movement integrates works out, for instance, running, significant yardwork and high-influence moving.

Strength preparing. Do strength preparing practices for all significant muscle bunches something like two times each week. Strength preparing can incorporate utilization of weight machines, your own body weight, weighty packs, obstruction tubing or opposition paddles in the water, or exercises, for example, rock climbing.

No enchanted slug

GREAT LIFE

Try not to seek dietary enhancements for help in consuming calories or shedding pounds. Items that case to accelerate digestion typically don't satisfy their cases. Some might cause awful secondary effects.

The U.S. Food and Medication Organization doesn't request confirmation that dietary enhancements are protected or that they work. Question the cases that are made. Continuously let your medical services suppliers in on about supplements you take.

There's no simple method for getting more fit. To take in less calories than you consume, the 2020-2025 Dietary Rules for Americans prescribes slicing 500 to 750 calories every day to lose 1 to 1.5 pounds (0.5 to 0.7 kilograms) seven days. Add more active work to get to

GREAT LIFE

your weight reduction objectives quicker and keep up with your weight reduction. A medical care supplier, like a specialist or enrolled dietitian, can assist you with investigating ways of shedding pounds.

Digestion and Maturing

As we age, metabolic cycles don't work as well as when we were more youthful. Our bodies don't process supplements from food as proficiently, which can cause blood glucose levels to be raised, especially after we devour a dinner. Also, anabolic cycles, for example, building muscle protein become less proficient, so it's harder to acquire bulk as we age. As a matter of fact, after age 50, grown-ups who don't practice lose a normal of 0.4 pounds of bulk every year.

GREAT LIFE

The Uplifting new

In any case, don't worry! There are various sound way of life systems that have been deductively demonstrated to balance a portion of these impacts. Integrate solid way of life ways of behaving into your everyday existence — the outcomes can be strong! Coming up next is a rundown of way of life systems and tips that have been demonstrated to influence the metabolic wellbeing of more seasoned grown-ups capably.

TIPS:

Continue To move

We as a whole know that customary high-impact work out (a.k.a. " cardio") is great for our wellbeing. Only 30

GREAT LIFE

minutes of basically moderate force work out, five days out of each week, improves for all intents and purposes all parts of metabolic wellbeing. In any case, what you can be sure of is that arising proof likewise recommends that decreasing the time you spend being stationary (a.k.a. sitting) and staying away from drawn out, nonstop inactive periods may likewise work on your digestion. Specialists report that while sitting is intruded on with short sessions (roughly five minutes) of one or the other strolling or standing, significant metabolic gamble factors, including blood glucose and insulin levels, improve — particularly following a feast (so don't simply sit subsequent to eating). No less than 30 minutes of moderate-power oxygen consuming

GREAT LIFE

action, no less than 5 days out of every week for a sum of 150 minutes Or possibly 25 minutes of lively vigorous movement no less than 3 days of the week for a sum of 75 minutes

Perform Muscle-Fortifying Exercises

Muscle-reinforcing exercises are alright for more established grown-ups and demonstrated to keep up with the respectability of muscle and bone, and further develop equilibrium, coordination and portability. Likewise, on the grounds that muscles are exceptionally metabolically dynamic, assembling and keeping up with sound bulk will assist with pushing your digestion along. These activities might try and diminish the signs and side effects of normal metabolic infections like

GREAT LIFE

diabetes and weight. Rules from the division of Wellbeing and Human Administrations suggest performing muscle-fortifying exercises, for example, lifting loads, obstruction band activities or body weight work out (like push-ups, sit-ups, and so on.) somewhere around two days out of every week.

Consume a Solid Eating routine Low in Handled Sugars

To fuel a sound digestion you ought to eat various supplement thick food varieties from every nutrition class. Supplement thick food sources are food sources that have a high supplement to calorie proportion like lean meats, vegetables and entire grains. You ought to restrict handled food varieties since they can be a subtle wellspring of added sugar, sodium and "void" calories

GREAT LIFE

— calories that convey restricted dietary benefit. Polishing off fiber-rich food varieties and drinking a lot of water may especially help metabolic wellbeing by supporting processing and bringing down glucose and cholesterol.

Pursue Sound Rest Routines

As we age, a decent night's rest can be difficult to find and this is thought to adversely influence significant parts of digestion, for example, blood glucose levels and insulin responsiveness. The purposes behind this are not completely perceived, yet specialists accept a mix of physiological, natural and conduct changes are at fault. Research shows that the accompanying tips can assist with advancing longer, more tranquil rest:

GREAT LIFE

Think Counteraction

It's never beyond any good time to profit from integrating significant wellbeing advancing ways of behaving into your life. Notwithstanding, that's what research demonstrates in the event that we start early, we are considerably more liable to keep a steady, sound body weight, which can be fundamental for safeguarding metabolic capability, decreasing our gamble for the majority ongoing circumstances and keeping up with useful freedom a ways into our brilliant years.

GREAT LIFE

GREAT LIFE

GREAT LIFE

CHAPTER THREE
SUPPORTING DIGESTION NORMALLY

Sustenance and Digestion

Energy is expected to incorporate particles into bigger macromolecules (like proteins), and to transform macromolecules into organelles and cells, which then, at that point, transform into tissues, organs, and organ frameworks, lastly into an organic entity. Appropriate sustenance gives the fundamental supplements to make the energy that upholds life's cycles. Your body assembles new macromolecules from the supplements in food.

Supplement and Energy Stream

GREAT LIFE

Energy is put away in a supplement's synthetic bonds. Energy comes from daylight, which plants catch and, through photosynthesis, use it to change carbon dioxide in the air into the particle glucose. At the point when the glucose bonds are broken, energy is delivered. Microorganisms, plants, and creatures (counting people) reap the energy in glucose through an organic cycle called cell breath. In this cycle oxygen is required and the substance energy of glucose is bit by bit delivered in a progression of synthetic responses. A portion of this energy is caught in the particle adenosine triphosphate (ATP) and some is lost as intensity. ATP can be involved when expected to drive compound responses in cells that require a contribution of energy.

GREAT LIFE

Cell breath requires oxygen (high-impact) and it is given as a result of photosynthesis. The results of cell breath are carbon dioxide (CO_2) and water, which plants use to direct photosynthesis once more. Consequently, carbon is continually cycling among plants and creatures. Plants reap energy from the sun and catch it in the particle glucose. People gather the energy in glucose and catch it into the atom ATP.

Eating is crucial for life. Large numbers of us hope to eating as a need, yet additionally a delight. You might have been advised since adolescence to begin the day with a decent breakfast to give you the energy to traverse the majority of the day. You in all probability have caught wind of the significance of a decent eating

GREAT LIFE

routine, with a lot of foods grown from the ground. Be that as it may, how might this all affect your body and the physiological cycles it completes every day? You really want to retain a scope of supplements so your cells have the structure blocks for metabolic cycles that discharge the energy for the cells to do their day to day positions, to fabricate new proteins, cells, and body parts, and to reuse materials in the cell.

This part will take you through a portion of the synthetic responses crucial for life, the amount of which is alluded to as digestion. The focal point of these conversations will be anabolic responses and catabolic responses. You will analyze the different synthetic responses that are essential to support life, including

GREAT LIFE

why you should have oxygen, how mitochondria move energy, and the significance of certain "metabolic" chemicals and nutrients.

Digestion differs, contingent upon age, orientation, movement level, fuel utilization, and lean weight. Your own metabolic rate vacillates over the course of life. By adjusting your eating routine and exercise routine, you can increment both lean weight and metabolic rate. Factors influencing digestion likewise assume significant parts in controlling bulk. Maturing is known to diminish the metabolic rate by as much as 5% each year. Also, on the grounds that men tend have more slender bulk then ladies, their basal metabolic rate (metabolic rate very still) is higher; accordingly, men

GREAT LIFE

will generally consume a bigger number of calories than ladies do. In conclusion, a person's inborn metabolic rate is an element of the proteins and compounds got from their hereditary foundation. In this way, your qualities assume a major part in your digestion. Regardless, every individual's body takes part in similar generally metabolic cycles.

Metabolic cycles are continually occurring in the body. Digestion is the amount of the substance responses that are all engaged with catabolism and anabolism. The responses overseeing the breakdown of food to get energy are called catabolic responses. Alternately, anabolic responses utilize the energy created by catabolic responses to combine bigger particles from

GREAT LIFE

more modest ones, for example, when the body structures proteins by hanging together amino acids. The two arrangements of responses are basic to keeping up with life.

Since catabolic responses produce energy and anabolic responses use energy, preferably, energy use would adjust the energy delivered. In the event that the net energy change is positive (catabolic responses discharge more energy than the anabolic responses use), then the body stores the overabundance energy by building fat atoms for long haul stockpiling. Then again, assuming the net energy change is negative (catabolic responses discharge less energy than anabolic responses use), the

GREAT LIFE

body utilizes put away energy to make up for the lack of energy delivered by catabolism.

Way of life Elements for Further developed Digestion

Your Metabolic Rate is impacted by numerous elements working in blend, including:

Body size - bigger grown-up bodies have seriously processing tissue and a bigger BMR.

Measure of slender muscle tissue - muscle consumes kilojoules quickly. Measure of muscle to fat ratio - fat cells are 'drowsy' and consume far less kilojoules than most different tissues and organs of the body. Crash slimming down, starving or fasting - eating too not many kilojoules urges the body to ease back the digestion to monitor energy. BMR can come around up to 15% and assuming slender muscle tissue is additionally lost, this further diminishes BMR.

Age - digestion eases back with age because of loss of muscle tissue, yet in addition because of hormonal and neurological changes.

Development - babies and kids have higher energy requests per unit of body weight because of the energy requests of development and the additional energy expected to keep up with their internal heat level.

Orientation - for the most part, men have quicker digestion systems since they will quite often be bigger.

GREAT LIFE

Hereditary inclination - your metabolic rate might be halfway settled by your qualities.

Hormonal and apprehensive controls - BMR is constrained by the anxious and hormonal frameworks. Hormonal uneven characters can impact how rapidly or gradually the body consumes kilojoules.

Natural temperature - in the event that temperature is extremely low or exceptionally high, the body needs to work harder to keep up with its generally expected internal heat level, which expands the BMR.

Contamination or sickness - BMR increments on the grounds that the body needs to work harder to assemble new tissues and to make an insusceptible reaction.

Measure of active work - diligent muscles need a lot of energy to consume. Normal activity increments bulk and helps the body to consume kilojoules at a quicker rate, in any event, when very still.

Drugs - like caffeine or nicotine, can expand the BMR.

Dietary lacks - for instance, an eating routine low in iodine diminishes thyroid capability and eases back the digestion.

GREAT LIFE

GREAT LIFE

CHAPTER FOUR
DIGESTION AND DIETARY METHODOLOGIES

Food sources that Help a Solid Digestion

Digestion is the cycle the body uses to change over food into the energy expected to make due and capability. Digestion frequently dials back because of things beyond our control, including maturing and hereditary qualities. Notwithstanding, there are a few sound changes you can make, such as eating right and working out, to assist with supporting your digestion. The better your body is, the better your digestion might work.

GREAT LIFE

Attempt these 12 quality food varieties, suggested by UnityPoint Wellbeing dietitian Allie Bohlman. Many are wealthy in fiber or protein, which can encourage you longer and backing weight reduction endeavors. Keep in mind, digestion is only one piece of the weight reduction puzzle.

Fish and Shellfish

Digestion Supporting Powers: Fish (salmon, fish, sardines and mackerel) are wealthy in omega-3 unsaturated fats and protein. Your body consumes somewhat a greater number of calories processing protein than fat and carbs.

GREAT LIFE

Tip: The American Heart Affiliation suggests individuals ought to eat greasy fish no less than two times each week. Could do without the flavor of fish? Take an omega-3 unsaturated fat (vegan amicable) or fish oil supplement.

Vegetables (Otherwise called beans)

Digestion Helping Powers: Vegetable is a general term used to depict the seeds of plants that are in cases. They incorporate high-protein dark bean, chickpeas and kidney beans.

Tip: Add vegetables in a simple and reasonable manner by putting canned beans on your shopping list. Assuming that you're watching salt admission, search for the low-sodium names. Take a stab at preparing beans in servings of mixed greens, soup recipes or pasta dishes.

Stew Peppers

Digestion Helping Powers: Hot peppers like stew peppers and jalapeños contain the compound capsaicin, which gives these vegetables their intensity. Capsaicin expands your body's inner temperature which briefly assists you with consuming more calories. Despite the fact that this could support your digestion, eating a greater amount of these will not fundamentally help your weight reduction.

GREAT LIFE

Tip: Barbecue, stuff, steam, heat or pan fried food a serving of peppers, or serve them crude to coordinate with low-fat plunges or curds.

Lean Meats

Digestion Supporting Powers: Chicken, turkey and other protein-stuffed lean meats take more energy for your body to separate than carb or fat-rich food varieties, in this way, consuming somewhat more calories during the stomach related process.

Tip: Cut back off any apparent excess from meat and poultry, including the skin. Low-fat cooking techniques incorporate searing, simmering, sautéing, barbecuing and baking.

GREAT LIFE

Low-Fat Milk

Digestion Supporting Powers: The calcium and vitamin D found in milk are fundamental for building thick bulk, which is significant for generally speaking wellbeing.

Tip: Add low-fat milk rather than water to oats, hot grains and consolidated cream soup. Request skim or 1% milk while requesting lattes and cappuccinos.

Broccoli

Digestion Helping Powers: Broccoli is an individual from the cruciferous vegetable family. It's known for its high water and fiber content, which is an extraordinary blend to assist you with feeling full.

GREAT LIFE

Tip: Eat broccoli steamed or simmered. Or on the other hand, appreciate it crude with a low-fat veggie plunge.

Lentils

Digestion Supporting Powers: Lentils are a kind of vegetable and are loaded with iron, magnesium and potassium. They are an incredible plant protein and fiber source with 8 grams of each. Lentils arrive in various tones including red, brown, green and yellow. All are similarly smart for you.

Tip: Grown-up ladies ought to get over two times how much iron as men. One cup of lentils gives around 35% of your everyday iron requirements.

Cereal

GREAT LIFE

Digestion Supporting Powers: This is a stalwart loaded with fiber that won't just assist you with enduring through the morning without hunger yet will dial back the arrival of sugar into your circulatory system.

Tip: Begin the day with a blistering bowl of cereal in the first part of the day or make for the time being oats the prior night in a bricklayer container for an in a hurry breakfast.

Berries

Digestion Supporting Powers: Berries, like blueberries and strawberries, are low in calories and high in fiber. Fiber advances generally speaking weight reduction by diminishing your craving.

GREAT LIFE

Tip: On the off chance that you can't find your #1 new berries, unsweetened frozen berries are a decent substitute during slow times of year and are comparably nutritious.

Almonds

Digestion Helping Powers: Almonds contain heaps of solid fats, fiber and protein, which is a mix that controls hunger.

Tip: Partake in a small bunch of almonds between feasts to stay away from undesirable bites or cleave them up for a crunchy salad clincher.

Low-Fat Curds

GREAT LIFE

Digestion Helping Powers: Curds is low in fat, low in carbs and high in protein, making it ideal for solid eaters.

Tip: Add a scoop of low-fat curds to a berry smoothie for a contemporary bend.

Tempeh

Digestion Helping Powers: Tempeh is an extraordinary protein substitute for meat in the event that you are searching for a veggie lover choice.

Tip: Take a stab at involving Tempeh in pan-sears, sandwiches, bowls or wraps.

Water

GREAT LIFE

Digestion Helping Powers: Water can smother your hunger and perhaps help your digestion for a short measure of time. Research proposes the more hydrated you are, the better capable your body is at pretty much all that from thinking to making exercise simpler.

Tip: Have a go at getting the day going with a glass of water or drink a glass before you eat your feasts. To decide how much water to drink each day, partition your weight down the middle. The number you get ought to be your fluid sum in ounces.

Remember about Your Muscles

Other than these smart dieting tips, one of the most amazing ways of accelerating your digestion is with

GREAT LIFE

weight or muscle reinforcing. Slender bulk expands your digestion. Muscle is metabolically dynamic, and that implies individuals with lean, solid bodies need more energy to work than individuals with a higher level of muscle versus fat. Make a point to chat with your primary care physician prior to starting any new exercise routine everyday practice.

Nourishing Enhancements for Metabolic Upgrade

Digestion is in a general sense influenced by specific nutrients and minerals, which help in energy creation and enzymatic responses. Guaranteeing a satisfactory admission of these supplements is key for keeping up with metabolic wellbeing.

GREAT LIFE

Nutrients and Their Effect on Digestion

My job is to feature the way in which explicit nutrients assume critical parts in changing over food into energy. B nutrients are especially critical in such manner.

Thiamin (B1) helps carb digestion, transforming sugars into energy.

Riboflavin (B2) is pivotal for oxidizing unsaturated fats and proteins.

Niacin (B3) aids DNA fix and stress reactions.

Pantothenic corrosive (B5) adds to the combination of coenzyme A, vital in using fats and starches.

GREAT LIFE

Pyridoxine (B6) is fundamental for amino corrosive digestion and red platelet creation.

Biotin (B7) helps in digestion of unsaturated fats, amino acids, and glucose.

Folate (B9) has an impact in DNA blend and fix, impacting cell development.

Cobalamin (B12) is fundamental for nerve capability and the union of DNA, and works with folate to deliver red platelets.

Every nutrient plays its own unmistakable part, yet on the whole they support a solid digestion by working with basic biochemical responses in energy creation.

Minerals Fundamental for Metabolic Cycles

GREAT LIFE

I'll presently zero in on the minerals imperative for metabolic capability. These include:

Iron: Fundamental for making energy from supplements, it is a part of hemoglobin in red platelets and myoglobin in muscle cells, conveying oxygen required for the ignition of fills in cell breath.

Calcium: Past its job in bone wellbeing, calcium is engaged with muscle constrictions and compound movement vital for digestion.

Magnesium: This mineral goes about as a cofactor for many protein frameworks that control different biochemical responses in the body, including energy creation, nerve capability, and muscle unwinding.

GREAT LIFE

Legitimate levels of these minerals are principal for guaranteeing our substantial cycles work without a hitch and really.

Dietary Contemplations for Upgrading Digestion

While expecting to upgrade digestion through diet, I center around unambiguous food decisions and the general equilibrium of the eating regimen. Reexamining eating examples can significantly affect metabolic productivity.

Compelling Food Decisions

I focus on food varieties that have been displayed to increment metabolic rate normally. Green tea is a perfect representation; it contains catechins and

GREAT LIFE

caffeine, which might help digestion marginally for a couple of hours. It's anything but a marvel arrangement, but instead a valuable decision to integrate into an eating regimen.

Proteins require more energy to process contrasted with fats and starches, along these lines including lean meats, dairy items, vegetables, and nuts can be helpful. I guarantee these are a reliable piece of my dinners.

Food Category   Examples

Proteins: Chicken, fish, tofu, eggs

Carbohydrates: Whole grains, yams

Fiber: Beans, broccoli, berries

GREAT LIFE

Consolidation of entire food starches, particularly those high in fiber, is critical. Fiber-rich food varieties, similar to organic products, vegetables, and entire grains, improve sensations of completion as well as assist with keeping a sound digestion.

Significance of Adjusted Diet on Digestion

I comprehend the significance of a decent eating routine for keeping a solid digestion. This equilibrium incorporates a blend of macronutrients - proteins, carbs, and fats - as well as micronutrients from a different scope of food varieties.

Guaranteeing my eating routine isn't vigorously slanted toward a specific macronutrient, I center around

GREAT LIFE

assortment. Balance in utilization of each macronutrient upholds metabolic wellbeing, alongside the consideration of a lot of vegetables and natural products for their nutrient, mineral, and fiber content.

Accentuation on sound digestion is definitely not a passing thought; it's a pledge to way of life changes. Checking my admission of macronutrients and picking digestion amicable food varieties assist me with keeping up with this equilibrium.

Way of life and Social Variables

In my investigation of how to support digestion, I've found that consolidating predictable active work and overseeing rest and stress are significant. These way of

GREAT LIFE

life decisions straightforwardly impact my metabolic rate and energy consumption.

Actual Activity and Digestion

My customary commitment to actual activity altogether expands my calorie consume. Strength preparing, specifically, constructs muscle, which consumes a greater number of calories than fat, even while very still:

High-impact work out: Helps in consuming countless calories in a meeting. For example, a lively 30-minute run can consume around 280-520 calories relying upon my weight and speed.

GREAT LIFE

Obstruction preparing: Upgrades bulk, which thusly raises my resting metabolic rate. Lifting loads for 20-30 minutes can consume between 90-126 calories.

Through predictable active work, I can work on my metabolic wellbeing and increment energy consumption.

Rest, Stress, and Metabolic Wellbeing

My rest examples and feelings of anxiety affect my digestion than I could understand. Satisfactory rest and stress decrease strategies are fundamental for keeping a sound digestion:

GREAT LIFE

Sleep: Holding back nothing hours out of every evening, as lacking rest can bring down my resting metabolic rate and increment hunger chemical levels.

Stress the executives: Rehearses like reflection and profound breathing activities can alleviate the antagonistic metabolic impacts of pressure, for example, the propensity to store instinctive fat.

Supplemental Guides for Digestion

I will cover two vital areas of interest: normal enhancements intended to improve metabolic rate and the job of regular concentrates in supporting digestion.

Normal Enhancements to Lift Digestion

GREAT LIFE

In the domain of digestion sponsor supplements, certain mixtures have acquired prevalence. Green tea extricate is habitually utilized, essentially because of its high grouping of epigallocatechin gallate (EGCG), a compound read up for expanding fat oxidation potential. Caffeine, one more common fixing, is notable for its thermogenic properties, which can upgrade calorie consume.

Furthermore, L-carnitine assumes a critical part by moving unsaturated fats into the cells for energy creation, hence it's normally found in supplements showcased to help a sound digestion. Probiotics likewise seem promising, as arising research

GREAT LIFE

recommends they might work on metabolic wellbeing by affecting stomach vegetation.

Green Tea Concentrate: Contains EGCG, which might support fat oxidation.

Caffeine: Invigorates thermogenesis and can increment metabolic rate.

L-carnitine: Aids unsaturated fat vehicle inside cells to support energy creation.

Probiotic: Upholds stomach wellbeing and may decidedly influence digestion.

Normal Concentrates and Their Adequacy

Going to normal concentrates as digestion helps, I view as a few essential. The zesty part of cayenne pepper, capsaicin, can briefly increment digestion through its thermogenic impact. This has started the consideration of cayenne or capsaicin supplements in digestion supporting items.

Moreover, extricates with cell reinforcement properties, as EGCG from green tea, support digestion as well as deal added medical advantages like superior heart wellbeing. It is essential to be careful that albeit these normal concentrates show potential, their belongings can change among people.

Cayenne Pepper: The capsaicin it contains can deliver a thermogenic outcome.

GREAT LIFE

EGCG: A cell reinforcement in green tea extricate that might uphold expanded digestion.

In examining these enhancements and regular concentrates, I expect to give a reasonable and genuine record of their apparent advantages in digestion help.

Wellbeing and Interview

In my quest for overseeing weight gain and helping digestion, I generally focus on wellbeing. Enhancements can offer likely advantages, however they accompany the requirement for alert. It's essential to counsel a medical care supplier prior to beginning any enhancement routine, particularly in the event that I have a condition like corpulence or on the other hand in the event that I'm taking drugs.

Medical care Supplier Direction

Appraisal: I look for direction to guarantee supplements don't struggle with my ongoing drugs.

Personalization: Counsel is customized to my singular wellbeing needs and objectives.

Figuring out Incidental effects

Cautiousness: I stay caution to any antagonistic responses that might show aftereffects.

GREAT LIFE

Reporting: Any bad side effects I experience ought to be expeditiously talked about with my medical services supplier.

Medicine Communications

Similarity: Enhancements can connect with prescriptions, changing their viability or hurting.

Review: I consistently survey my drug with a medical services supplier while adding enhancements to my routine.

Proof Based Decisions

By following these pathways, I assume responsibility for my wellbeing with certainty and informed alert. Going with insightful supplementation decisions turns

GREAT LIFE

out to be essential for a more extensive procedure to deal with my weight and further develop metabolic wellbeing really and securely.

GREAT LIFE

CHAPTER FIVE
DEFEATING NORMAL METABOLIC DIFFICULTIES

Digestion and Hormonal Equilibrium

Chemicals are substance couriers that significantly affect your psychological, physical, and profound wellbeing. For example, they assume a significant part in controlling your hunger, weight, and mind-set.

Your body commonly delivers the exact measure of every chemical required for different cycles to keep you solid. Nonetheless, stationary ways of life and Western dietary examples might influence your hormonal climate. Likewise, levels of specific chemicals decline

GREAT LIFE

with age, and certain individuals experience a more emotional diminishing than others.

A nutritious eating routine and other sound way of life propensities might assist with working on your hormonal wellbeing and permit you to feel and play out your best.

Eat sufficient protein at each feast

It is critical to Consume sufficient measures of protein.

Besides the fact that protein gives fundamental amino acids that your body can't make all alone, yet your body additionally needs it to deliver protein-determined chemicals — otherwise called peptide chemicals. Your endocrine organs make these chemicals from amino acids. Peptide chemicals assume a vital part in controlling numerous physiological cycles, like development, energy digestion, hunger, stress, and propagation.

For instance, protein admission impacts chemicals that control craving and food consumption, conveying data about energy status to your mind. Research has shown that eating protein diminishes the yearning chemical ghrelin and animates the development of chemicals that assist you with feeling full, including peptide YY (PYY) and glucagon-like peptide-1 (GLP-1).

One 3-month concentrate on in 156 youngsters with corpulence corresponded a high protein breakfast with expanded PYY and GLP-1 levels, which brought about

GREAT LIFE

weight reduction because of expanded sensations of completion. Specialists suggest eating at least 15-30 grams of protein for every feast. You can do this by including high protein food varieties like eggs, chicken bosom, lentils, or fish at every feast.

Take part in standard activity

Actual work unequivocally impacts hormonal wellbeing. Beside further developing blood stream to your muscles, practice increments chemical receptor responsiveness, implying that it upgrades the conveyance of supplements and chemical signs.

GREAT LIFE

A significant advantage of activity is its capacity to diminish insulin levels and increment insulin responsiveness.

Insulin is a chemical that permits cells to take up sugar from your circulatory system to use for energy. Nonetheless, in the event that you have a condition called insulin obstruction, your phones may not successfully respond to insulin. This condition is a gamble factor for diabetes, weight, and coronary illness.

In any case, while certain specialists actually banter whether the enhancements come from practice itself or from getting more fit or fat, proof shows that normal activity might further develop insulin obstruction autonomously of body weight or fat mass decrease.

GREAT LIFE

Many sorts of active work have been found to assist with forestalling insulin obstruction, including stop and go aerobic exercise, strength preparing , and cardio.

Being actually dynamic may likewise assist with supporting degrees of muscle-keeping up with chemicals that decay with age, like testosterone, IGF-1, DHEA, and development chemical (HGH).

For individuals who can't perform incredible activity, even ordinary strolling might increment key chemical levels, possibly further developing strength and personal satisfaction.

Keep a moderate weight

GREAT LIFE

Weight gain is straightforwardly connected with hormonal uneven characters that might prompt complexities in insulin responsiveness and regenerative wellbeing. Corpulence is firmly connected with the advancement of insulin obstruction, while losing overabundance weight is connected to upgrades in insulin opposition and decreased chance of diabetes and coronary illness.

Heftiness is likewise connected with hypogonadism, a decrease or nonattendance of chemical discharge from the testicles or ovaries. As a matter of fact, this condition is one of the most significant hormonal difficulties of weight in individuals doled out male upon entering the world.

GREAT LIFE

This implies heftiness is emphatically connected with lower levels of the regenerative chemical testosterone in individuals doled out male upon entering the world and contributes an absence of ovulation in individuals relegated female upon entering the world, the two of which are normal reasons for fruitlessness.

Regardless, studies show that weight reduction might switch this condition. Eating inside your very own calorie reach can assist you with keeping up with hormonal equilibrium and a moderate weight.

Deal with your stomach wellbeing

Your stomach contains in excess of 100 trillion well disposed microbes, which produce various metabolites

"

GREAT LIFE

that might influence chemical wellbeing both decidedly and adversely.

Your stomach microbiome directs chemicals by balancing insulin obstruction and sensations of completion . For instance, when your stomach microbiome matures fiber, it delivers short-chain unsaturated fats (SCFAs) like acetic acid derivation, propionate, and butyrate.

Acetic acid derivation and butyrate may help weight the executives by expanding calorie consuming and consequently assist with forestalling insulin opposition.Acetic acid derivation and butyrate may likewise manage sensations of completion by expanding the totality chemicals GLP-1 and PYY.

GREAT LIFE

Curiously, concentrates on in rodents show that corpulence might change the creation of the stomach microbiome to advance insulin opposition and aggravation.

Moreover, lipopolysaccharides (LPS) — parts of specific microscopic organisms in your stomach microbiome — may build your gamble of insulin obstruction. Individuals with weight appear to have more elevated levels of coursing LPS.

Here are a few hints to keep up with solid stomach microscopic organisms which may likewise assist you with keeping a sound chemical equilibrium.

Bring down your sugar consumption

GREAT LIFE

Limiting added sugar admission might be instrumental in enhancing chemical capability and staying away from stoutness, diabetes, and different illnesses. The basic sugar fructose is available in many sorts of sugar, containing up to 43% of honey, half of refined table sugar , 55% of high fructose corn syrup, and 90% of agave.

Likewise, sugar-improved refreshments are the essential wellspring of added sugars in the Western eating regimen, and fructose is normally utilized monetarily in soda pops, natural product squeeze, and game and caffeinated drinks.

Fructose consumption has expanded dramatically in the US since around 1980, and concentrates reliably show

GREAT LIFE

that eating added sugar advances insulin obstruction —

at any rate some of which are free of absolute calorie

admission or weight gain, Long haul fructose admission

has been connected to interruptions of the stomach

microbiome, which might prompt other hormonal

lopsided characteristics.

In addition, fructose might neglect to animate the

creation of the completion chemical leptin, prompting

diminished calorie consuming and expanded weight

gain. Thusly, diminishing your admission of sweet

beverages — and different wellsprings of added sugar

— may further develop chemical wellbeing.

Attempt pressure decrease strategies

GREAT LIFE

Stress hurts your chemicals in more ways than one.

The chemical cortisol is known as the pressure chemical since it assists your body with adapting to long haul pressure. Your body's reaction to stretch enacts a fountain of occasions that prompts cortisol creation. When the stressor has passed, the reaction normally closes.

Nonetheless, ongoing pressure debilitates the criticism components that assist with returning your hormonal frameworks to typical.

In this way, constant pressure causes cortisol levels to stay raised , which animates craving and expands your admission of sweet and high fat food sources. Thusly,

GREAT LIFE

this might prompt over the top calorie admission and corpulence. What's more, high cortisol levels animate gluconeogenesis — the development of glucose from non-starch sources — which might cause insulin obstruction.

Prominently, research demonstrates the way that you can bring down your cortisol levels by taking part in pressure decrease strategies like contemplation, yoga, and paying attention to loosening up music.

Attempt to give no less than 5 minutes out of each day to these exercises.

Consume solid fats

GREAT LIFE

Remembering great regular fats for your eating routine might assist with diminishing insulin opposition and craving. Medium-chain fatty substances (MCTs) are special fats that are less inclined to be put away in fat tissue and bound to be taken up straight by your liver for guaranteed use as energy, advancing expanded calorie consuming.

MCTs are likewise less inclined to advance insulin obstruction.

Besides, sound fats, for example, omega-3sTrusted Source assist with expanding insulin responsiveness by diminishing aggravation and favorable to provocative markers.

GREAT LIFE

These solid fats are found in unadulterated MCT oil, avocados, almonds, peanuts, macadamia nuts, hazelnuts, greasy fish, and olive and coconut oils.

Get predictable, excellent rest

Regardless of how nutritious your eating regimen or how predictable your work-out daily practice, getting sufficient supportive rest is pivotal for ideal wellbeing. Unfortunate rest is connected to lopsided characteristics in a large number, including insulin, cortisol, leptin, ghrelin, and HGH.

For example, not in the least dozes hardship disable insulin responsiveness, yet unfortunate rest is related

GREAT LIFE

with a 24-hour expansion in cortisol levels, which might prompt insulin obstruction.

As a matter of fact, one little concentrate in 14 sound grown-ups found that 5 evenings of rest limitation diminished insulin responsiveness by 25%.

Besides, concentrates reliably show that lack of sleep brings about expanded ghrelin and diminished leptin levels. In addition, your mind needs continuous rest to go through every one of the five phases of each rest cycle. This is particularly significant for the arrival of development chemical, which happens primarily around evening time during profound rest.

GREAT LIFE

To keep up with ideal hormonal equilibrium, hold back nothing 7 hours of great rest each evening.

Follow a high fiber diet

Fiber is vital for a sound eating routine.

Albeit dissolvable fiber will in general create the most grounded outcomes on craving by expanding totality chemicals, insoluble fiber may likewise assume a part.

Your stomach microbiome ages dissolvable fiber in your colon, creating SCFAs that animate the arrival of the totality chemicals PYY and GLP-1.

GREAT LIFE

Reasonable Tips for Regular Metabolic Wellbeing

If you have any desire to help your wellbeing and prosperity, there are a lot of regular and home solutions for browse, going from staying away from roasted meats and added sugars to rehearsing contemplation. With regards to understanding what's sound, even qualified specialists frequently appear to hold contradicting conclusions. This can make it hard to sort out how you ought to really be streamlining your wellbeing.

However, regardless of the multitude of conflicts, various health tips are all around upheld.

GREAT LIFE

The following are 10 wellbeing and sustenance tips that depend on logical proof.

Limit sweet beverages

Sweet beverages like soft drinks, natural product squeezes, and improved teas are the essential wellspring of added sugar in the American eating routine

Sugar-improved refreshments are additionally extraordinarily unsafe for kids, as they can contribute not exclusively to corpulence in youngsters yet additionally to conditions that normally don't create until adulthood, similar to type 2 diabetes, hypertension, and non-alcoholic greasy liver sickness

GREAT LIFE

Better options include:

water

unsweetened teas

shining water

espresso

Eat nuts and seeds

Certain individuals stay away from nuts since they are high in fat. Nonetheless, nuts and seeds are staggeringly nutritious. They are loaded with protein, fiber, and different nutrients and minerals Nuts might assist you with getting in shape and decrease the gamble of creating type 2 diabetes and coronary illness

GREAT LIFE

Furthermore, one enormous observational review noticed that a low admission of nuts and seeds was possibly connected to an expanded gamble of death from coronary illness, stroke, or type 2 diabetes

Keep away from super handled food sources

Super handled food varieties (UPFs) are food sources containing fixings that are fundamentally altered from their unique structure. They frequently contain added substances like added sugar, exceptionally refined oil, salt, additives, counterfeit sugars, tones, and flavors also

Models include:

nibble cakes

GREAT LIFE

cheap food

frozen feasts

bundled treats

chips

UPFs are exceptionally attractive, meaning they are effectively overeaten, and enact reward-related districts in the cerebrum, which can prompt abundance calorie utilization and weight gain. Concentrates on demonstrate the way that counts calories high in super handled food can add to heftiness, type 2 diabetes, coronary illness, and other persistent circumstances

Try not to fear espresso

GREAT LIFE

Regardless of some contention over it, espresso is stacked with medical advantages.

It's wealthy in cell reinforcements, and a few examinations have connected espresso admission to life span and a decreased gamble of type 2 diabetes, Parkinson's and Alzheimer's sicknesses, and various different diseases. In any case, it's ideal to consume espresso and any caffeine-based things with some restraint. Over the top caffeine admission might prompt medical problems like sleep deprivation and heart palpitations. To appreciate espresso in a protected and sound manner, keep your admission to under 4 cups each day and stay away from unhealthy, high-sugar added substances like improved half and half.

GREAT LIFE

Eat greasy fish

Fish is an incredible wellspring of great protein and solid fat. This is especially valid for greasy fish, for example, salmon, which is stacked with mitigating omega-3 unsaturated fats and different supplements

Get sufficient rest

The significance of getting sufficient quality rest couldn't possibly be more significant.

Unfortunate rest can drive insulin opposition, can upset your hunger chemicals, and lessen your physical and mental exhibition

In addition, unfortunate rest is one of the most grounded individual gamble factors for weight gain

GREAT LIFE

and stoutness. Individuals who don't get sufficient rest will more often than not pursue food decisions that are higher in fat, sugar, and calories, possibly prompting undesirable weight gain

Feed your stomach microbes

The microorganisms in your stomach, altogether called the stomach microbiota, are unimaginably significant for in general wellbeing.

A disturbance in stomach microbes is connected to a few persistent illnesses, including corpulence and a bunch of stomach related issues

Great ways of further developing stomach wellbeing incorporate eating matured food varieties like yogurt and sauerkraut, taking probiotic supplements — when shown — and eating a lot of fiber. Strikingly, fiber fills in as a prebiotic, or a food hotspot for your stomach microorganisms

Remain hydrated

Hydration is a significant and frequently neglected marker of wellbeing. Remaining hydrated guarantees that your body is working ideally and that your blood volume is adequate Drinking water is the most effective way to remain hydrated, as it's liberated from calories, sugar, and added substances.

GREAT LIFE

Despite the fact that there's no limited sum that everybody needs each day, expect to drink enough so your thirst is satisfactorily extinguished

Try not to eat intensely burned meats

Meat can be a nutritious and sound piece of your eating regimen. It's very high in protein and a rich wellspring of enhancements

In any case, issues happen when meat is scorched or consumed. This singing can prompt the development of hurtful mixtures that might build your gamble for specific diseases

At the point when you cook meat, do whatever it takes not to singe or consume it. Furthermore limit your

GREAT LIFE

utilization of red and handled meats like lunch meats and bacon as these are connected to by and large disease chance and colon malignant growth risk

Keep away from splendid lights before rest

At the point when you're presented to brilliant lights — which contain blue light frequencies — at night, it might upset your creation of the rest chemical melatonin.

Far to assist with decreasing your blue light openness is to wear blue light impeding glasses — particularly in the event that you utilize a PC or other computerized screen for significant stretches of time — and to stay

GREAT LIFE

away from computerized evaluates for 30 minutes to an hour prior hitting the sack.

This can assist your body with bettering produce melatonin normally as night advances, assisting you with dozing better.

GREAT LIFE

CHAPTER SIX
ACCOMPLISHING
BOUNDLESS WELLBEING

Comprehensive Ways to deal with Health

In the event that the term comprehensive health evokes pictures of smoky rooms and purple gems, you're in good company. All encompassing health has become pretty sensationalized.

In any case, the "charm" term mirrors a modern perspective on individuals as the entirety of their encounters, not only one name or thought. Also, assuming we comprehend that individuals are perplexing, that implies that we comprehend there's no "one" meaning of health, by the same token. As a rule,

GREAT LIFE

individuals mean one of two things when they discuss all encompassing wellbeing. The term is many times utilized as a shorthand for elective medication. For instance, on the off chance that somebody had a clinical conclusion, they might search for "normal" approaches to treating the disease. This would be "comprehensive medication."

The more extensive meaning of comprehensive health utilizes the strict importance of "all encompassing." That is, it characterizes wellbeing as the reliance of a few elements of wellbeing. The entire individual, subsequently, isn't well except if they're well in each everyday issue — not simply actual wellbeing. While specialists banter which regions ought to be

GREAT LIFE

remembered for comprehensive wellbeing, most concur that it envelops mental, profound, and actual wellbeing.

This is the way every one of these areas connects with generally health:

Mental health

Mental prosperity — and mental wellness — is essential to by and large wellbeing. Mental wellness permits us to speak with others, think fundamentally, and settle on choices effortlessly. A solid brain can learn and develop, and can remain present at the time. Poor mental wellness is related with diminished versatility and protection from stress.

Actual wellbeing

GREAT LIFE

Actual prosperity is at times considered being liberated from sickness. Be that as it may, just "not being debilitated" doesn't actually make for much personal satisfaction. Then again, there are people who live with constant infection who feel imperative and well. Actual wellbeing incorporates energy, adaptability, strength, wellness, rest, and nourishment.

Profound health

Being sincerely sound effects your relationship with yourself as well as other people. Profound health decides how you decipher unpleasant circumstances and your capacity to direct feelings. It additionally works on your capacity to request help and sit with awkward feelings. Taking into account that self

GREAT LIFE

destruction positions as a main source of death in the US, mental and profound wellbeing are obviously basic to general wellbeing.

Profound wellbeing

Profound wellbeing alludes to your association with an option that could be bigger than yourself. Individuals who are in a deep sense solid can track down reason and significance throughout everyday life. They feel more persuaded, are stronger, and have a feeling of their spot on the planet. Those with unfortunate otherworldly wellbeing will quite often encounter existential emergencies.

Social health

GREAT LIFE

Social prosperity is driven by a feeling of having a place. Taking part in associations, investing energy with loved ones, and feeling associated with others are all essential for social wellbeing. Specialists have found that those with solid informal organizations live longer, better lives.

Word related health

We spend a critical part of our lives at work, so it makes sense that what we feel when we're there means for our other lives. Word related wellbeing remembers finding happiness and satisfaction for the work that we do. It additionally implies feeling like you have valuable chances to develop and foster inside your vocation.

GREAT LIFE

Monetary health

While monetary wellbeing is excluded from the NWI's model, numerous other health experts feel that it merits its own classification. A 2020 review observed that monetary pressure was related with lower efficiency, spirit, and expanded pressure. Individuals with poor monetary wellbeing feel that they need command over their pay and costs. They stress over their capacity to deal with crises and have lower confidence.

Blissful individual stands-in-garden-comprehensive wellbeing

Best practices to accomplish comprehensive health

GREAT LIFE

There are vast ways of making all encompassing wellbeing arrangements — and there's no "correct" reply. As you become more mindful of the manner in which various parts of your life meet, you might observe that there are times when one region turns out to be a higher priority than others. In some cases, an answer or movement will lose the strength of its positive effect. Remain liberal and empathetic as you foster this new, entire individual way to deal with prosperity.

The accompanying ideas are incredible ways of beginning seeing the effect that one part of health has on the others. Pick the one that feels the simplest or generally effective for you to execute, or use it as a

GREAT LIFE

leaping off highlight make an all encompassing methodology that works for you.

Integrate rest into your day

It very well may be hard to stand by when you realize you have a ton to achieve. Notwithstanding, rest makes you more compelling, more imaginative, and more joyful. Getting sufficient rest — and rest, yet every one of the seven unique sorts of rest — is basic to your all encompassing wellbeing. Have a go at setting a clock to remind yourself to enjoy reprieves. Utilize your time away from work to accomplish something that re-energizes you inventively and profoundly.

Work with a mentor

GREAT LIFE

Some of the time, it's difficult to perceive what various components of wellbeing might be meaning for different parts of your life. Working with a health expert, specialist, or mentor can give knowledge concerning what changes will have the greatest effect on your general prosperity.

For instance, assuming you're feeling disappointed working, you might expect that this is on the grounds that you're not being genuinely made up for your work. That might be valid, yet the subsequent effect on your monetary, social, and close to home prosperity might have more to do with how you as of now feel. Life or wellbeing instructing can assist you with sorting out the

GREAT LIFE

most ideal way to explore your conditions, decide the main driver, and accomplish your objectives.

Grasp the association among physical and mental wellness

Actual prosperity immensely affects our psychological and profound prosperity. Dealing with your actual wellbeing by getting sufficient rest, practicing routinely, and eating great can work on your temperament and mental capacity. You can consolidate different elements of all encompassing health too, such as hitting an exercise class with a companion or running a 5K to help a reason you trust in. Taking care of oneself practices like needle therapy, chiropractic care, and care are

GREAT LIFE

additionally great ways of sustaining the entire body, brain, and soul.

Support your connections

Social wellbeing, especially fabricating connections that motivate us, assists us with fostering a feeling of having a place. We develop how we might interpret ourselves — and in numerous ways, our confidence — by how we are seen by everyone around us. Concentrate intently on building connections in light of shared objectives, support, and common regard. These connections will affect how you feel, what you eat, and even how much cash you make.

Remain receptive

GREAT LIFE

Incredulous about taking a yoga class, contemplating, or seeking a Reiki treatment? At any rate, attempt it. A long time back, individuals murmured that you could "get" an evil spirit from being excessively near someone else. That sounds pretty out there — except if you believe it to be a simple hypothesis of irresistible illness. Since we don't completely comprehend how something functions isn't motivation not to attempt it. What's more, on the off chance that it cheers you up, we are in general for it.

Accomplish something that you love

Shuffling work, individual connections, and expert improvement doesn't allow for the sake of entertainment — yet you must focus on it at any rate.

GREAT LIFE

Accomplishing something that you love only for it keeps your innovativeness streaming. Time spent accomplishing something fun very corresponds to how proficient you are in your work time. It just so happens, the more you are at play, the more you are working.

Regardless of the normal misinterpretation, all encompassing health isn't about sage and gems (despite the fact that assuming that is your thing, we unquestionably won't pass judgment). About understanding individuals as diverse creatures have rich, nuanced encounters. These everyday issues cross and cover to make the aggregate of how we feel out of nowhere. Adopting an entire individual strategy to wellbeing is vital to assisting people with living their most joyful, best, and most satisfying lives.

Mind-Body Association and Digestion

At the point when I ponder my reality, I'm fast to think about my actual body and my normal exercises. Then, I contemplate past encounters and future objectives, communications with others, and afterward the manners in which I have adjusted to explore my environmental elements.

Society has a fascinating relationship with the actual space that we each possess and like numerous things throughout everyday life, pretty much contrasted with your ongoing plot might appear to be ideal at some random time. Without a doubt, bodies alone give a

GREAT LIFE

design however the mind boggling processes that happen inside these vessels makes every one of us exceptional individual creatures. On the off chance that you have at any point considered how we can occupy such little room at the end of the day yet be so plentiful then you are perfectly located.

Each body experiences a progression of cell exercises to keep it alive which we frequently allude to as the digestion. The many-sided cycles of digestion are generally subject to the manners by which we sustain our bodies through nourishment, circadian synchronizing, development, care, and social availability.

GREAT LIFE

One of the directing variables of digestion is the dietary benefit of the food sources we devour. Assimilation starts with the admission of supplements that are separated and changed over into particles fundamental for protein amalgamation, cell fix, and detoxification prior to finishing off with disposal of waste. Routine utilization of plants like organic products, vegetables, entire grains, beans, nuts, and seeds have been connected to longer life expectancies in a few networks across the world. On the other hand, eating a supplement less eating regimen comprising of exceptionally handled food varieties isn't ideal for the stomach microflora and can thusly prompt diminished

GREAT LIFE

energy, discouraged temperament, and can add to infection of different organ frameworks.

Digestion is personally attached to a natural cycle known as circadian musicality. While considering everyday schedules you might envision the dawn, espresso, work liabilities, eating dinners, tasks, active work, watching your number one show, and rest. What you might not have thought of, nonetheless, is that these everyday customs are more interconnected than they could appear. For example, our bodies wake normally through an outpouring of chemical signals that happen when the sun rises. Additionally, when the sun sets, melatonin is delivered to assist us with getting to rest. Circadian synchronizing is an all encompassing

GREAT LIFE

practice that perceives a few metabolic cycles are more proficient during waking hours and others adjust better to a resting state. This regular beat is likewise attached to hunger and the need to consume energy.

This takes us back to the primary resource with supplements which is our gastrointestinal system and the amazing organization inside it known as the stomach microbiome. The trillions of life forms (microscopic organisms, growths, protozoa, and infections) that make up this vegetation are impacted by hereditary qualities, climate, diet, fiber consumption, hurtful substances, and meds. In any case, microorganisms assume a part in resistant capability, impact metabolic wellbeing and disease risk, influence

GREAT LIFE

pressure reaction and mental working, and add to our neurochemistry and ways of behaving. Every individual microbiota is extraordinary and can be either advantageous to generally speaking wellbeing or, when sub-standard, can increment risk for sickness.

The connection between the stomach microbiome and mind wellbeing has turned into an intricate subject of interest. Organisms in the gastrointestinal lot have been displayed to impact synapses like serotonin and dopamine. They have additionally been attached to ways of behaving related with torment, feeling, social cooperations, and food admission. Expanding the quantity of gainful microorganisms in the stomach

GREAT LIFE

through dietary change can possibly modify the stomach microbiome and improve mental capability.

Development is one more part of our reality that is additionally connected to neurochemistry and our circadian chemicals. The American School of Cardiology suggests no less than 150 minutes of activity each week for ideal cardiovascular wellbeing. This device has for quite some time been utilized in the administration of neuropsychiatric problems, to keep up with mental wellbeing, and might actually be utilized to postpone the beginning of neurodegenerative cycles. All the more as of late, moderate activity following a feast was displayed to diminish blood glucose levels which can bring down the gamble for type 2 diabetes. Besides, bunch exercise can add to a feeling of having a place and social network that has likewise been displayed to increment life expectancy.

The cross-over of development and care is powerful. Take yoga or kendo for example that carry out body developments, breathing, and a thoughtful encounter. Care exercises animate neuronal pathways that diminishing pressure and emphatically impact state of mind. For this reason a movement as straightforward as recording Three Beneficial Things (there's an application for that) every day can develop appreciation, increment hopefulness, further develop rest, and lift joy.

GREAT LIFE

In impression of what it genuinely means to exist, I think it is critical to perceive that we are far beyond the actual space we possess. Sustenance, development, care rehearses, and our associations with others influence our wellbeing on a cell level. We have various biochemical and neurochemical pathways that make us every one of a kind. It is the interconnectedness of our bodies and our psyches that permit us to interface with our surroundings and with others to support our prosperity and develop life span.

GREAT LIFE

GREAT LIFE

CONCLUSION

Pushing Ahead: Supporting Great Energy

Go to the store, and you'll see a huge number of nutrients, spices, and different enhancements promoted as energy sponsors. Some are even added to sodas and different food sources. In any case, there's almost no logical proof that energy promoters like ginseng, guarana, and chromium picolinate really work. Fortunately, you can improve your normal energy levels by doing things. The following are nine hints:

Control pressure

Stress-incited feelings consume enormous measures of energy. Chatting with a companion or relative, joining a

GREAT LIFE

care group, or seeing a psychotherapist can all assist with diffusing pressure. Unwinding treatments like reflection, self-entrancing, yoga, and jujitsu are additionally viable apparatuses for decreasing pressure.

Safeguard yourself from the harm of constant aggravation.

Science has demonstrated that persistent, second rate irritation can transform into a quiet executioner that adds to cardiovas-cular sickness, disease, type 2 diabetes and different circumstances. Get straightforward tips to battle irritation and remain solid -- from Harvard Clinical School specialists.

Relieve your burden

GREAT LIFE

One of the fundamental purposes behind weakness is exhaust. Exhaust can incorporate proficient, family, and social commitments. Attempt to smooth out your rundown of "must-do" exercises. Put forth your boundaries regarding the main errands. Pare down those that are less significant. Think about requesting additional assistance at work, if fundamental.

Work out

Practice nearly ensures that you'll rest all the more adequately. It likewise gives your cells more energy to consume and flows oxygen. Also, practicing can prompt higher mind dopamine levels, which raises temperament. While strolling, quit slacking occasionally to get additional medical advantages.

GREAT LIFE

Try not to smoke

You realize smoking undermines your wellbeing. Regardless, you may not understand that smoking truly diverts your energy by causing a resting issue. The nicotine in tobacco is an energizer, so it speeds the pulse, raises circulatory strain, and animates mind wave movement related with attentiveness, making it harder to nod off. What's more, when you in all actuality do nod off, its habit-forming power can kick in and stir you with desires.

Limit your rest

Assuming you figure you might be sleepless, have a go at getting less rest. This exhortation might sound odd

GREAT LIFE

yet deciding how much rest you really need can lessen the time you spend in bed not dozing. This cycle makes it simpler to nod off and advances more peaceful rest over the long haul. This is the method for getting it going:

Try not to rest during the day.

The principal night, hit the sack later than ordinary and get only four hours of rest.

Assuming you feel that you rested soundly during that four-hour time span, add another 15-30 minutes of rest the following evening.

GREAT LIFE

However long you're resting adequately the whole time you're sleeping, gradually continue to include rest progressive evenings.

Eat for energy

Eating food varieties with a low glycemic record — whose sugars are retained gradually — may assist you with keeping away from the slack in energy that regularly happens subsequent to eating immediately consumed sugars or refined starches. Food varieties with a low glycemic file incorporate entire grains, high-fiber vegetables, nuts, and solid oils like olive oil. By and large, high-sugar food varieties have the most elevated glycemic records. Proteins and fats have glycemic files that are near nothing.

GREAT LIFE

Use caffeine for your potential benefit

Caffeine helps increment readiness, so having some espresso can assist with honing your brain. However, to get the stimulating impacts of caffeine, you need to reasonably utilize it. It can cause sleep deprivation, particularly when consumed in huge sums or after 2 p.m.

Limit liquor

One of the most incredible supports against the midafternoon droop is to try not to drink liquor at lunch. The calming impact of liquor is areas of strength for particularly noontime. Likewise, stay away from a five o'clock mixed drink to have energy at night. On the

GREAT LIFE

off chance that you will drink, do as such with some restraint when you wouldn't fret having your energy wind down.

Hydrate

What's the principal supplement that has been shown to redesign execution for everything aside from the most mentioning persistence works out? It's not a few expensive games drink. It's water. In the event that your body is shy of liquids, one of the main signs is a sensation of weariness.